AF510095

IBS Low-FODMAP Made Simple

A 4-Week Guide to Find Triggers, Master Reintroduction & Build Your Personal Plan (Meal Plan + Recipes)

mf

Disclaimer

This guide is provided for informational and educational purposes only and should not be interpreted as medical, nutritional, or professional advice. The author is not a licensed physician, nurse, dietitian, or mental health provider. Reading this guide does not establish a patient–provider relationship of any kind.

Always seek the guidance of a qualified healthcare professional before starting, changing, or discontinuing any supplement, diet, or lifestyle program. If you are pregnant, breastfeeding, managing a chronic medical condition, or taking prescription medications, consult your physician or pharmacist before considering any product mentioned in this guide.

The author and publisher make no representations or warranties regarding accuracy, applicability, fitness, or completeness of the information contained herein. While every effort has been made to ensure scientific accuracy and currency, medical knowledge and research evolve continually. Readers are responsible for verifying information and making decisions in consultation with licensed professionals.

Use of this guide and any information contained within it is at your own risk. The author and publisher disclaim all liability for any loss, injury, or adverse outcome that may result from the use or misuse of this material.

No supplement, diet, or practice discussed in this text is intended to diagnose, treat, cure, or prevent any disease. No outcomes or benefits are guaranteed.

Product names, supplement formulations, diet frameworks, and trademarks mentioned are the property of their respective owners and are used for identification only. Any images or illustrations that appear in related materials are licensed stock or educational placeholders.

Table of Contents

Introduction

Irritable bowel syndrome (IBS) is a common digestive disorder that affects a significant proportion of adults worldwide. Characterized by symptoms such as abdominal pain, bloating, and irregular bowel habits, IBS can have a considerable impact on daily quality of life. Estimates suggest that millions of adults contend with IBS, though the condition often remains undiagnosed or misdiagnosed due to the variability of symptoms and their overlap with other gastrointestinal issues. Understanding IBS is the first step toward managing it, and dietary approaches have become a central focus for both clinicians and those living with the disorder.

One aspect of IBS that has gained increased scientific attention is how certain carbohydrates, specifically a group called FODMAPs can trigger or worsen symptoms. FODMAP stands for Fermentable Oligo-, Di-, Mono-saccharides, and Polyols. These are short-chain carbohydrates found in a wide range of foods, including some fruits, vegetables, grains, and dairy products. For individuals with IBS, FODMAPs can be poorly absorbed in the intestine, leading to excessive fermentation by gut bacteria. This process produces gas and draws water into the bowel, resulting in symptoms like bloating, abdominal discomfort, and altered bowel movements. The link between FODMAPs and IBS symptoms is now well recognized, providing a tangible target for dietary intervention.

The clinical rationale for employing a Low-FODMAP diet to manage IBS is anchored in solid scientific investigation. Studies have shown that systematically restricting high-FODMAP foods can significantly reduce IBS symptoms in the majority of patients, often within just a few weeks. The Low-FODMAP diet is not a fad or a form of unnecessary restriction, but a structured method for identifying and managing individual food triggers. The initial phase typically involves minimizing intake of all high-FODMAP foods to achieve symptom relief, followed by a careful reintroduction phase to pinpoint which specific FODMAPs a person can tolerate and in what amounts.

A structured 4-week Low-FODMAP program offers multiple benefits. First, it provides a timeframe that is long enough to see meaningful symptom improvement, yet short enough to avoid unnecessary long-term restriction of beneficial foods. By following a weekly progression elimination, symptom tracking, reintroduction, and personalization individuals can gain valuable insights into their own tolerances and dietary needs. This approach not only promotes digestive comfort but also supports psychological well-being by restoring a sense of predictability around meals and social situations.

In this guide, you will discover:

- A step-by-step four-week process for implementing the Low-FODMAP diet safely and effectively
- Core knowledge about IBS and FODMAPs
- Guidance on preparation, elimination, detailed symptom monitoring, and systematic food reintroduction
- Strategies for creating a customized maintenance plan
- Sample recipes, meal planning aids, troubleshooting tips, and advice for adapting the diet to your unique lifestyle

The intended outcome is not just short-term symptom relief, but lasting control over IBS through a flexible, evidence-based eating approach.

Whether you're newly diagnosed or have struggled with IBS for years, this comprehensive guide is designed to empower you with the tools and understanding needed to reclaim your digestive health. With a clear structure and actionable insights, you can look forward to discovering your own path to greater comfort and confidence at the table.

IBS Basics and the Role of Gut Health

Key IBS symptoms and diagnostic criteria

Irritable Bowel Syndrome (IBS) is a functional gastrointestinal disorder marked by symptoms that fluctuate over time. Its central feature is recurring or persistent abdominal pain, usually related to defecation or a change in the frequency or appearance of stool. Other common issues include bloating, excess gas, diarrhea, constipation, or combinations of these.

Diagnosis relies primarily on the Rome criteria: abdominal pain averaging at least one day per week over the past three months, plus two or more of the following: pain related to defecation, changes in stool frequency, or changes in stool form. Importantly, IBS is diagnosed only after excluding other potential causes, such as inflammatory bowel disease or celiac disease.

For many, IBS is disruptive, impacting daily routines, work, social life, and psychological health. The routine pain, urgency, and bloating can prompt people to avoid activities or foods, further diminishing quality of life.

A defining aspect of IBS is its unpredictability. The symptom pattern can shift both from person to person and from day to day. Some experience flares only occasionally; others deal with symptoms multiple times a week. Symptom triggers can include stress, dietary changes, hormonal shifts, or environmental factors. Because IBS symptoms overlap with other conditions and are often intermittent, diagnosis and management can be challenging. Personal tracking of symptoms and triggers, however, provides a vital foundation for effective self-management.

The Gut-Brain Axis in IBS

IBS is not solely a gastrointestinal issue; it stems from interactions between the gut and the brain, governed by the gut-brain axis. This axis is a two-way communication network connecting the brain, the enteric nervous system (sometimes called the "second brain" in the gut), the immune system, and gut microbiota.

Communication occurs via nervous, hormonal, and immune signals that affect gut movement, sensation, secretions, and immune responses. People with IBS often have visceral ***hypersensitivity***, meaning normal stretching of the bowel from gas or stool causes disproportionate pain or discomfort, even with no visible inflammation or structural abnormality.

Stress and psychological distress can heighten this gut sensitivity, creating a feedback loop where each exacerbates the other. In turn, gut symptoms can intensify anxiety or depression. This explains the value of stress management strategies such as mindfulness, gentle exercise, or cognitive behavioral therapy in IBS care.

The gut-brain axis also highlights how foods exert effects beyond basic nutrition; they can influence brain chemistry, gut movements, and the makeup of the gut microbiota. Disruptions in these communication networks, triggered by stress, illness, or dietary shifts, can provoke IBS symptoms.

Evidence-Based Risk Factors for Symptom Flare-Ups

While IBS symptom flares might sometimes appear to arise without warning, research has identified several well-established risk factors that can contribute to these episodes. Understanding these factors can empower individuals to manage their symptoms more effectively. The key risk factors include the following:

1. ***Diet***: What you eat plays a significant role in triggering IBS symptoms. Foods high in FODMAPs short-chain carbohydrates that are poorly absorbed by the small intestine—are especially problematic. These fermentable carbs can draw excess water into the gut and are broken down by bacteria, leading to increased

gas production, abdominal pain, and bloating. Examples of high-FODMAP foods include onions, garlic, beans, certain fruits, and dairy products.

2. ***Stress and Psychological Factors***: Emotional wellbeing greatly influences gut health. High-stress events, whether negative (such as illness or job loss) or positive (such as moving to a new home or getting married), can precipitate or exacerbate gut symptoms. This is primarily due to communication between the gut and the brain, known as the gut-brain axis. Many people with IBS observe that their symptoms intensify during periods of anxiety or emotional distress and improve when they are feeling calm and relaxed.
3. ***Changes in Routine***: Disruptions to daily routines can also serve as triggers. Factors such as travel, illness, changes in sleep patterns, or even alterations in work schedules can upset the gut's normal functioning. These changes may lead to irregular eating habits or sleeping patterns, both of which can contribute to symptom flare-ups.
4. ***Medications and Hormonal Fluctuations***: Certain medications, including antibiotics or pain relievers, may irritate the digestive system. Additionally, hormonal changes, such as those that occur during the menstrual cycle, can influence IBS symptoms, making some people more susceptible to flares at specific times of the month.

5. ***Physical Inactivity***: A sedentary lifestyle can worsen IBS symptoms. Regular physical activity is known to support healthy digestion and reduce stress, making it an important component of symptom management.

These risk factors often interact with one another. For example, consuming a high-FODMAP meal after a night of poor sleep and high stress is more likely to provoke a flare than eating the same meal during a restful, calm period. This complex interplay highlights the value of a holistic management approach that addresses not just diet, but also stress management, sleep quality, physical activity, and emotional wellbeing.

Importance of Individualized Dietary Interventions

Irritable Bowel Syndrome (IBS) presents uniquely in each individual, with symptom patterns and dietary triggers varying widely. As a result, broad, one-size-fits-all dietary recommendations often fail to address the specific needs of those affected. Experts emphasize the value of personalized dietary interventions that consider each person's symptoms, food preferences, and nutritional requirements. A tailored plan can more effectively support symptom management and promote overall wellness.

1. The low-FODMAP diet exemplifies a personalized approach. Instead of eliminating entire food groups

indefinitely, this strategy introduces a phased process: first, most high-FODMAP foods are temporarily removed during an elimination phase; next, foods are systematically reintroduced to identify which ones cause symptoms.

2. This step-by-step method safeguards against the risks associated with indiscriminate dietary restriction. Potential consequences such as nutritional deficiencies, excessive weight loss, or social isolation due to limited food choices can be minimized.
3. Systematic reintroduction of foods enables individuals to discover which foods are well-tolerated, allowing for a more varied and enjoyable diet. Unnecessary avoidance of foods is reduced, supporting both nutritional adequacy and quality of life.
4. Maintaining a detailed food and symptom diary throughout this process can provide valuable insights. Tracking meals alongside symptom patterns helps clarify which foods may be true triggers and which are safe to include.
5. Involving a knowledgeable dietitian is highly recommended, particularly for those with additional health concerns or dietary restrictions. Professional guidance ensures that the individualized plan remains nutritionally balanced and sustainable over time.

Individualized dietary interventions are key to effectively managing IBS symptoms and improving overall well-being.

By adopting a personalized approach with professional support, individuals can achieve better symptom control while maintaining a balanced and enjoyable diet.

Connection Between Gut Microbiota and FODMAP Intake

Research highlights a close, dynamic relationship between gut microbiota, the trillions of microbes in our intestines and the foods we ingest. This connection is especially relevant in IBS.

FODMAPs act as substrates for certain gut bacteria. When these carbohydrates reach the colon undigested, bacteria ferment them, producing gases such as hydrogen, methane, and carbon dioxide, which can trigger bloating, pain, and altered bowel habits. Gut microbes also influence production of short-chain fatty acids, immune responses, and gut sensitivity.

People with IBS often have a gut microbiota composition distinct from those without IBS. This imbalance, or dysbiosis, may cause heightened sensitivity to particular FODMAPs, or modify how and how quickly fermentation occurs. Consequently, two people may react very differently to the same food based on their unique microbial profile.

Reducing FODMAP intake can quickly alter the gut microbiota and frequently alleviates symptoms. However, long-term FODMAP restriction may decrease beneficial gut bacteria and their metabolites, so the elimination phase should be brief, with gradual reintroduction to preserve microbial diversity and gut health.

Balancing symptom relief with nurturing a healthy microbiota is essential to contemporary IBS dietary management. As microbiota, diet, and symptoms continually interact, the ideal dietary plan is one that is revisited and adjusted as your situation and tolerance change.

Practical Application: Linking the Science to Your Everyday Life

Applying IBS and low-FODMAP knowledge in daily life turns understanding into progress:

1. ***Track Your Symptoms***: Keep a diary of food intake, symptoms, bowel habits, stress, and sleep. Patterns will often reveal which foods or situations worsen symptoms.
2. ***Recognize Non-Food Triggers***: Non-dietary factors like stress, anxiety, lack of sleep, or disrupted routines can be as significant as food. Addressing these can improve symptom control as much as dietary modification.
3. ***Embrace Personalization***: Your symptom triggers are personal. What is fine for one person may cause problems for another. The low-FODMAP method is

about creating a tailored, flexible diet based on your own experiences and reactions.

4. ***Collaborate with Professionals***: Dietitians and healthcare providers are valuable resources, especially during the elimination and reintroduction phases of a low-FODMAP approach. If you have complex dietary or health needs (such as other food intolerances or specific eating preferences), professional support helps ensure symptom improvement and nutritional adequacy.
5. ***Focus on Gut Health Long-Term***: Short-term symptom relief is important, but maintaining gut health remains a central goal. Eat the widest range of well-tolerated fruits, vegetables, whole grains, and fermented foods as possible. Avoid unnecessarily prolonged restrictive diets.

With this understanding, you are equipped to begin a dietary journey that is grounded in scientific evidence and tailored to your unique needs. Upcoming chapters will guide you step by step through the low-FODMAP process, troubleshooting, and building a sustainable long-term management plan for IBS.

Successful IBS management aims to do more than just reduce symptoms; it seeks to improve overall quality of life by balancing control of IBS, nutritional sufficiency, and enjoyment of food. By understanding your own version of IBS, the role of the gut-brain axis, symptom triggers, and the relationship between diet and gut microbiota, you'll be empowered to make informed decisions and adjust your strategies as needed. Whether your experience with IBS is recent or long-standing, this knowledge offers a solid base to regain confidence in managing your health and making choices that work best for you.

Science of FODMAPs Explained

Definition and Classification of FODMAPs

FODMAPs are a specific group of carbohydrates found widely in our everyday foods, and their physiological impact has become central to modern dietary management of IBS symptoms. The term "FODMAP" stands for Fermentable Oligosaccharides, Disaccharides, Monosaccharides, and Polyols.

Each of these is a type of short-chain carbohydrate that shares two defining features: they are poorly absorbed in the small intestine and are rapidly fermented by bacteria in the colon. Collectively, these characteristics make FODMAPs highly relevant to digestive health, especially for individuals with heightened gastrointestinal sensitivity.

To better understand the science behind this, let's break down each component:

- ***Oligosaccharides***: These include fructans and galacto-oligosaccharides, commonly found in foods like wheat, onions, and legumes.

- ***Disaccharides***: Primarily lactose, the sugar present in milk and many dairy products.
- ***Monosaccharides***: Namely, fructose in excess of glucose, as often occurs in apples, honey, and high-fructose corn syrup.
- ***Polyols***: Sugar alcohols such as sorbitol and mannitol, present in certain fruits and vegetables, as well as many sugar-free products.

Not everyone reacts in the same way to these compounds. While FODMAPs are present in many healthy foods, their interaction with the gut plays a unique and sometimes problematic role for individuals with sensitive digestion. When these carbohydrates are consumed, their poor absorption draws extra water into the small intestine.

Moving onward to the colon, the rapid fermentation process begins, leading to the production of gas and other byproducts. For many people, especially those managing IBS, this sequence triggers discomfort, pain, and a range of disruptive gastrointestinal symptoms.

List of Common High and Low-FODMAP Foods

A practical understanding of which foods contain high versus low levels of FODMAPs is essential for anyone managing IBS or starting a low-FODMAP diet. Familiar foods can contain surprising amounts, so learning to distinguish between high- and low-FODMAP choices forms the foundation of successful symptom management.

Common high-FODMAP foods include:

- ***Wheat-based products*** like bread, pasta, and cereals.
- ***Certain fruits***: apples, pears, cherries, mangoes, and watermelons.
- ***Dairy products***: milk, soft cheeses, ice cream, and yogurts (due to lactose).
- ***Garlic and onions***, both extremely high in fructans.
- ***Legumes and pulses***: lentils, chickpeas, beans.
- ***Sweeteners*** such as honey, agave nectar, and sugar alcohols (sorbitol, mannitol, xylitol).

In contrast, there are many naturally low-FODMAP foods across all food groups, allowing for healthy eating without deprivation:

- ***Grains***: rice, oats, quinoa, and gluten-free breads made with suitable flours.
- ***Fruits***: bananas, blueberries, strawberries, oranges, grapes, and pineapples.
- ***Vegetables***: carrots, potatoes, zucchini, spinach, and bell peppers.
- ***Proteins***: plain cooked meats, fish, eggs, and firm tofu.
- ***Most nuts and seeds*** (with the exception of pistachios and cashews).

- ***Lactose-free dairy products or hard cheeses***, such as cheddar or Swiss, which have most of the lactose removed.

This distinction is not absolute; portion size matters greatly. Some foods are low-FODMAP in small portions but trigger symptoms when consumed in greater amounts. Paying attention to recommended serving sizes is a vital part of implementing the diet effectively.

Mechanisms by Which FODMAPs Cause IBS Symptoms

To understand why FODMAPs are so significant in the context of IBS, it's helpful to appreciate their exact mechanisms of action within the digestive tract. After consumption, FODMAPs progress through the gastrointestinal system largely undigested until they reach the colon. In individuals with IBS or a sensitive gut, the following processes are especially relevant:

1. **Water Retention in the Small Intestine:**

   Because FODMAPs are poorly absorbed, they attract and hold onto water as they pass through the small intestine. This can create an osmotic effect, increasing water content inside the gut and sometimes leading to loose stools, urgency, or diarrhea-like symptoms.

2. **Fermentation and Gas Production in the Colon:**

   Upon reaching the large intestine, FODMAPs are quickly fermented by gut bacteria. This fermentation produces gases such as hydrogen, methane, and carbon dioxide. While everyone's gut produces some gas, those with IBS often experience heightened sensitivity to this expansion of their intestines, resulting in bloating, discomfort, visible distention, and cramping.

3. **Motility and Nerve Responses:**

   The above processes combine with increased sensitivity of the gut's internal nerves. Many people with IBS have guts that react more intensely to stretching and chemical signals, amplifying the perception of pain and unrest. This visceral hypersensitivity means that what is an average volume of gas for many can be particularly uncomfortable, even debilitating, for some individuals.

It is not necessarily the FODMAPs themselves that are problematic for all people, but rather the body's exaggerated reaction especially when pre-existing IBS or digestive sensitivity is present. This forms the scientific underpinning of using a structured low-FODMAP diet as a method to identify and control triggers.

Variability in FODMAP Tolerance

It's essential to recognize that FODMAP tolerance varies significantly from person to person. While the mechanisms by which they cause symptoms are well-understood, not every individual with IBS is sensitive to each category of FODMAP to the same extent. Some may be highly reactive to fructans but handle lactose without difficulty, whereas others might only experience symptoms when consuming excess polyols.

Several factors influence this variability:

- ***Gut bacterial composition***: The population and type of bacteria residing in the colon dictate the speed and type of fermentation that occurs, and thus the volume and type of gas produced.
- ***Degree of gut sensitivity***: People with more pronounced visceral sensitivity or low pain thresholds are more reactive to ordinary distention or water shifts.
- ***Underlying digestive abilities***: For example, many people from certain genetic backgrounds can digest lactose into adulthood, while others lose this capability and develop lactose intolerance.
- ***Portion size is another critical variable***. Some people can enjoy small serves of high-FODMAP foods without discomfort, but will experience symptoms when portions increase. The low-FODMAP diet is therefore not intended as an all-or-nothing elimination.

Instead, it is a tool to discover personal thresholds and tailor eating habits accordingly.

The reason for this individualized approach is twofold. First, unnecessarily strict dietary restriction can decrease quality of life and potentially impact gut health by limiting fiber and diversity of nutrients. Second, understanding one's personal tolerance opens the door to a more satisfying and sustainable eating pattern after the initial elimination and reintroduction phases.

Tools for identifying FODMAP contents in foods

Navigating the wide range of packaged goods, homemade dishes, and restaurant meals can be daunting when you're working to avoid high-FODMAP triggers. Fortunately, there are several helpful strategies and tools for identifying which foods to choose (or avoid).

The following approaches can assist in identifying FODMAP contents:

1. **Food Lists and Guides:**

   Reliable, up-to-date lists of high- and low-FODMAP foods are foundational. Organizations with expertise in FODMAP research, such as Monash University, offer detailed databases and charts. These help clarify where foods fall on the spectrum, including specific portion sizes considered safe or problematic.

2. **Reading Ingredient Labels:**

   Many packaged foods and restaurant items contain "hidden" FODMAPs in the form of additives, sweeteners, or small quantities of wheat, garlic, or onion powder. Learning to scrutinize ingredient lists for triggers like high-fructose corn syrup, inulin, chicory root, sugar alcohols (ending in -ol), and various gums is critical. While some names may be unfamiliar at first, developing a habit of checking labels empowers you to maintain control over your diet in diverse eating environments.

3. **Mobile Apps:**

   There are validated smartphone apps, some supported by academic or clinical research teams, that allow you to search foods and check FODMAP content on the go. These tools can be especially useful when grocery shopping or eating out. Many include traffic-light systems (green/yellow/red) or searchable lists of both whole foods and commercial products, as well as tips for portion control and recipe adaptation.

4. **Meal Planning Resources:**

   Structured meal planning templates and recipe collections designed specifically for low-FODMAP compliance can take the guesswork out of daily eating. Comprehensive meal plans detail safe foods across breakfast, lunch, dinner, and snacks. For example, low-FODMAP meal planning guides suggest portion-controlled servings of rice, gluten-free oats, meats, safe fruits (such as strawberries and grapes), and vegetables like spinach and carrots, all while avoiding common high-FODMAP pitfalls.

5. **Professional Support:**

   While tools and guides are helpful, consulting with a registered dietitian knowledgeable in FODMAPs can provide individualized advice tailored to your needs. A dietitian can help interpret food lists, suggest substitutions, and ensure nutritional adequacy especially when managing complex or co-existing dietary conditions.

The science behind FODMAPs is ongoing. Regularly updated resources are valuable, as scientific testing can shift foods between high- and low-FODMAP categories as new information emerges. Set reminders to periodically check your resource guides or app databases for the latest recommendations.

Understanding the science behind FODMAPs is a crucial first step for anyone seeking to use dietary changes to manage IBS. FODMAPs, those fermentable short-chain carbohydrates, are a diverse group of food components found in both common staples and specialty foods. Their potential to trigger digestive distress through water retention, fermentation, and gas production underscores why they have become a major focus for managing IBS symptoms.

Learning to differentiate high- from low-FODMAP foods, appreciating the personalized nature of FODMAP tolerance, and employing practical tools for food identification equips you for the journey ahead. The low-FODMAP diet is not about permanent restriction or eliminating entire food groups forever; it's about empowering you to discover your unique triggers and create an individualized, nutritionally adequate way of eating.

The upcoming chapters will offer practical steps to put this science into action starting with preparation, symptom tracking, and the elimination phase that form the backbone of the 4-week low-FODMAP approach. Armed with a clear understanding of the foundational science, you are well-positioned to make meaningful improvements in digestive comfort and overall wellbeing.

Preparing for the Low-FODMAP Journey

Starting a Low-FODMAP diet is more than a food change; it's an adjustment in mindset, routines, and habits. Solid preparation before the elimination phase increases confidence, reduces unexpected hurdles, and lets you meaningfully track your IBS symptom progress. This chapter covers setting expectations, symptom assessment, kitchen readiness, supportive environments, and the use of food symptom diaries.

Setting Realistic Expectations for the 4-Week Plan

Anticipating rapid relief is understandable with frustrating IBS symptoms, but success comes from balancing hope with realism. Some notice significant symptom improvements within two to six weeks with careful FODMAP restriction; for others, changes can be slow and gradual, especially as the gut adjusts.

Four weeks strikes a balance between allowing time for the gut to settle and avoiding excessive restriction. Consider this process an experiment with your body, not a rigid prescription. This mindset reduces pressure and encourages learning.

The first week typically brings a learning curve with new foods and ingredient awareness. Slip-ups, like accidentally eating high-FODMAP foods, are common, especially at the beginning, and should be viewed as normal parts of learning not failure. Even strict adherence cannot guarantee full IBS symptom resolution, as IBS triggers extend beyond FODMAPs. Still, many people do observe reduced bloating, abdominal pain, or altered bowel habits in the early weeks.

The Low-FODMAP process goes beyond elimination. After four weeks, gradually reintroducing different FODMAP groups clarifies your personal sensitivities, so your diet can expand while still avoiding trigger foods. Expect gradual progress, some challenges, and the need for patience and monitoring. Having these expectations prepares you for short-term improvement and long-term sustainability.

Assessing Baseline Symptoms and Triggers

Before making changes, record your current symptom patterns without altering your routine. This “baseline” provides a point of comparison for later, so you can accurately evaluate the diet’s effect. Common IBS symptoms include bloating, abdominal pain or discomfort, gas, diarrhea, constipation, or a mix.

To assess baseline:

- For at least three days, log everything you eat and drink, noting times and approximate portions.
- Record your key digestive symptoms, their timing, and severity (e.g., none, mild, moderate, severe).
- Observe correlations: Does bloating reliably follow certain meals or times of day? Are there nonfood triggers such as stress or inactivity?

This initial diary helps you target meals or situations most likely associated with symptoms as the plan progresses. It also prevents misattributing day-to-day symptom variability to diet alone.

Identifying both typical symptom patterns and known personal triggers allows more informed choices throughout the four weeks and supports better troubleshooting if symptoms persist.

Kitchen and Grocery Checklist for Low-FODMAP Compliance

Preparation is key for successful implementation. Organize your kitchen so low-FODMAP choices are easy and accidental high-FODMAP intake is minimized.

1. **Pantry and Kitchen Audit**
   - Survey your cupboards, fridge, and freezer for high-FODMAP foods: regular wheat bread, many cereals and pastas, processed foods containing onion or garlic, sauces, and high-lactose dairy.
   - Store these either separately or at the back, labeling them if needed especially when sharing a household with others not on the plan.

2. **Stocking Up on Low-FODMAP Staples**

   Essentials include:

   - Gluten-free breads, crackers, and flours (as wheat/rye are high-FODMAP in usual servings)
   - Lactose-free dairy or plant-based milks (almond, oat—if tolerated)
   - Plain meats, fish, eggs, tofu
   - Low-FODMAP fruits: firm bananas, oranges, grapes, blueberries, kiwifruit
   - Low-FODMAP vegetables: carrots, zucchini, spinach, tomatoes, potatoes
   - Grains: rice, quinoa, polenta
   - Olive oil and limited other plant oils
   - Safe herbs, chives, spices (avoid garlic/onion)
   - Canned lentils or chickpeas (rinsed, and only in modest, specified portions)

3. **Grocery Shopping Tips**
    - Prepare a list and stick to it to avoid impulsive, unsuitable purchases.
    - Read ingredient labels carefully; onion, garlic, and certain sweeteners (high-fructose corn syrup, honey, sorbitol) often hide in packaged foods.
    - Many processed and "healthy" products use wheat flour or milk powder check ingredients.
    - Use certified low-FODMAP food lists or specially designed recipes to aid selection and meal planning.

Batch-cooking and freezing low-FODMAP meals or snacks helps avoid high-FODMAP processed foods during busy weeks.

Designing Supportive Eating Spaces

Your environment influences your progress. Arrange spaces like your kitchen, dining area, and workplace to support your goals.

Suggestions include:

- Designate prep/cooking areas for low-FODMAP meals, helpful if sharing a kitchen with others.
- Store essentials where you see and reach them easily.

- Keep tools like measuring cups and kitchen scales on hand for portion accuracy.
- Plan meals and snacks in advance, using templates or pre-filled lists to ease daily decision-making.
- Bring meals with you in quality containers for work or school lunches.
- Prepare emergency low-FODMAP snacks to keep in your bag, car, or desk for unexpected hunger.
- Communicate with household members or frequent dining companions about your dietary needs to foster understanding and minimize social friction.

For social events, review menus ahead, call venues to check ingredient options, or bring your own suitable dishes. These tactics help you stay engaged socially without risking dietary setbacks.

Role of Food Symptom Diaries in Tracking

A detailed food and symptom diary is the most powerful tool to monitor your progress. It helps connect specific foods, timings, and portion sizes with any symptoms—noting patterns more precisely than memory allows.

Benefits:

- Increases awareness of actual intake versus intentions.
- Helps identify hidden FODMAP sources or overlooked eating habits.

- Lets you and your clinician make data-based decisions for next steps.
- Offers clear evidence of progress and clarifies which foods are triggers.

Keeping an Effective Diary

- Choose the format (notebook, app, spreadsheet) you'll consistently use.
- Log every meal and snack: time, description, estimated portions.
- Note any symptoms, recording type, timing, severity, and duration.
- Record relevant factors: stress, exercise, menstrual cycle, sleep quality these can affect IBS symptoms along with diet.

Example:

Breakfast (8:00 AM): Oatmeal with almond milk, sliced kiwifruit, 1 boiled egg

Symptoms: Mild bloating at 8:45 AM, gone by 10:00 AM

Lunch (12:30 PM): Grilled chicken, quinoa salad (spinach, carrots, olive oil & lemon), orange

Symptoms: None

Snacks (3:30 PM): Rice cakes with peanut butter

Symptoms: None

Specifics about portions, preparation, and brands increase diary usefulness, especially during elimination and reintroduction stages.

Troubleshooting Diary Use

- If you miss an entry, skip the guilt and just resume as soon as possible.
- Be as honest and specific as you can; accuracy beats perfection.
- Logging a few details daily is better than nothing.
- Bring your diary to appointments with your dietitian, as recall often misses key trends.

These preparation steps change a daunting dietary overhaul into manageable, confidence-building actions. By calibrating your expectations, mapping symptoms, preparing your kitchen, designing supportive environments, and recording your experience, you equip yourself for a smoother FODMAP journey.

No two people experience IBS or dietary responses identically. With preparation, consistent self-monitoring, and adaptability, you'll be ready to meet challenges and recognize your progress.

With your kitchen ready, eating areas organized, and baseline recorded, you're set to begin Week 1: the Elimination Phase. The step-by-step foundation you've built here will help make the coming weeks less confusing and more reassuring.

Week 1 – Low-FODMAP Elimination Phase

This first week marks a crucial transition: moving from preparation to action. The Low-FODMAP Elimination Phase is your opportunity to give your digestive system a rest from foods most likely to trigger IBS symptoms. This week is all about precision, attentiveness, and laying the groundwork for a successful dietary reset.

Structured Approach to Complete FODMAP Removal

The foundation of the elimination phase is the meticulous removal of high-FODMAP foods from your meals. FODMAPs (Fermentable Oligosaccharides, Disaccharides, Monosaccharides, and Polyols) are present in a variety of everyday foods, from wheat bread and apples to garlic, onions, and honey. For those with IBS, these compounds can cause excessive fermentation and water movement in the intestines, leading to pain, bloating, and unpredictable bowel habits.

To ensure a meaningful trial, it is necessary to remove all significant sources of FODMAPs for a short, finite window typically two to six weeks, with the first week setting the tone for careful attention to details. Unlike many restrictive diets, the Low-FODMAP approach is not about permanent deprivation but about working with your body's unique responses to food.

Take a structured approach:

1. Begin with a master list of high-FODMAP foods to exclude. This list typically includes wheat-based products, most dairy with lactose, certain fruits (like apples, pears, and stone fruits), legumes, and sweeteners such as honey and high-fructose corn syrup.
2. Use a credible, up-to-date resource such as those from Monash University or dedicated FODMAP support apps to check specific foods and FODMAP thresholds.
3. Plan all meals and snacks ahead for the week to minimize hunger-driven choices or accidental lapses.

By rigorously following an elimination plan, you provide the clearest possible "signal" when tracking your IBS symptoms. Lapses, substitution slip-ups, or guesswork can muddy results and prolong the process.

Daily Sample Meal Plan with Portion Sizes

Sticking to a Low-FODMAP menu can feel daunting in the first week, especially if your previous diet included many FODMAP-containing staples. Careful meal planning, clear portion guidance, and a simple, repetitive structure for days 1–7 can simplify things and reduce anxiety.

Below is a balanced, practical sample meal plan for one day during the elimination phase. All foods and portion sizes are selected for low-FODMAP content, and you are encouraged to repeat or rotate similar combinations throughout the week.

Breakfast:

- Scrambled eggs (2) with spinach (1 cup, raw) sautéed in olive oil (1 tsp)
- 1 slice gluten-free toast (check that there are no added high-FODMAP ingredients)
- 1 small orange (no larger than 130g)
- Black coffee or plain tea

Mid-Morning Snack:

- 1 medium firm banana (choose unripe to just-ripe for lowest FODMAPs)
- Handful (30g) of almonds (limit to ≤10 nuts to stay low-FODMAP)

Lunch:

- Grilled chicken breast (100g) salad with mixed lettuce (1 cup), cucumber (½ cup), carrot (½ cup), and a lemon-olive oil vinaigrette
- ¼ cup cooked quinoa
- Lemon water

Afternoon Snack:

Lactose-free yogurt (150g) topped with shredded coconut (1 tbsp) and strawberries (5 medium berries)

Dinner:

- Baked salmon fillet (120g)
- Steamed zucchini (½ cup) and carrots (½ cup)
- ½ cup cooked rice (white or brown)
- Sprinkling of fresh herbs and olive oil

Evening Snack:

- Rice cakes (2) with peanut butter (1 tbsp total)
- Herbal tea

Keep in mind that even low-FODMAP foods have recommended portion sizes. Exceeding these may make a meal moderate- or high-FODMAP. For example, a handful of almonds is low-FODMAP, but a full cup is not; the same principle applies to certain fruits and snack foods.

Feel free to swap out lean proteins (chicken, fish, firm tofu), low-FODMAP vegetables (bell peppers, tomatoes, carrots, lettuce), and permitted grains or starches (rice, oats, polenta) to suit your palate. The key is consistency and clarity. Record every ingredient if you are unsure.

Strategies to Avoid Accidental FODMAP Intake

Despite your best efforts, accidental FODMAP intake is possible, especially when eating unfamiliar foods, using seasonings, or trying new packaged products. A successful elimination phase relies on not just food selection, but vigilance in all aspects of shopping, prepping, and eating.

Some best practices:

- Read ingredient lists for hidden sources: Watch for "inulin," "fructooligosaccharides," "wheat flour," "honey," or "high-fructose corn syrup" all can introduce FODMAPs.
- Use simple, whole-food recipes during elimination. Embrace homemade dressings, sauces, and snacks to retain full control.
- When eating out (if unavoidable), opt for plain grilled meats or fish, steamed rice, and simply prepared vegetables. Request olive oil and lemon on the side, avoid sauces, and specify no garlic or onion.

- Be cautious with condiments and processed foods: Many contain high-FODMAP sugars or stabilizers. Choose plain, minimally processed options.

Watch for "natural flavors," "spices," or "vegetable powders" on ingredient lists, as these can contain onion or garlic extracts.

Consider batch cooking for the week and storing meals in labeled containers to reduce temptation and streamline daily decisions. If you find yourself unsure about a food, opt to skip it or substitute it with a clearly low-FODMAP alternative until you can confirm its status.

Cross-contamination in shared kitchens can also trip up progress. Use separate utensils and cutting boards if roommates or family members cook with high-FODMAP ingredients.

Monitoring for Changes in Symptom Patterns

A central goal of week one is to observe, record, and understand in real time the connection between what you eat and how you feel. Removing FODMAPs is not only about minimizing symptoms but about providing a "clean slate" to watch for changes in bloating, pain, bowel frequency, and urgency.

Best practices for monitoring include:

- At the end of each day, record main meals, snacks, and all beverage choices in your food diary.
- Use a simple scale (e.g., 0 = no symptoms, 10 = worst ever) to rate pain, bloating, stool consistency, and frequency. Note times of day.
- Document changes in energy, mood, and sleep, as these often improve alongside gut symptoms.
- Record any accidental FODMAP exposures however minor and the body's response over the next 24–48 hours.

Be patient with the process. It is common for improvements to appear by the end of week one, but for some, clear improvements may take longer.. Track trends, not isolated "good" or "bad" days. The key is to identify sustained reductions in symptom intensity or frequency, rather than seeking total elimination of symptoms immediately.

Adaptation: If a symptom spikes unexpectedly, revisit ingredient labels, preparation steps, dining-out history, and cross-contamination risks for clues. Use setbacks as data not as reasons to give up.

Adapting Elimination to Individual Food Preferences

A common concern with the Low-FODMAP elimination phase is that it may feel boring, repetitive, or incompatible with cultural preferences. The truth is, this phase can and should be tailored for taste, texture, and variety, within the limits of low-FODMAP guidelines.

Here's how to customize the elimination experience:

1. ***Make a list of your favorite low-FODMAP foods***, including proteins (eggs, poultry, tofu, fish), vegetables (carrots, zucchini, bell peppers, spinach), fruits (oranges, kiwi, strawberries), grains (oats, rice, quinoa), and lactose-free or plant-based dairy alternatives.
2. ***Use herbs (parsley, basil, rosemary)***, infused oils, and permitted spices to enhance flavor without adding FODMAPs.
3. ***Prepare culturally relevant meals*** by adapting traditional recipes: for example, swap wheat noodles for rice noodles in stir-fries, use canned lentils (drained and rinsed, maximum ¼ cup) in Mediterranean salads, or try gluten-free pastas made with corn or rice.
4. ***Explore simple, IBS-friendly recipes*** designed for the Low-FODMAP diet such as frittatas with safe vegetables, stir-fries using appropriate sauces, and homemade low-FODMAP soups.
5. ***Mix and match breakfast*** options try overnight oats (made with lactose-free milk and chia seeds), smoothies with allowed fruits, or savory rice porridge.

Take advantage of community-sourced resources, like cookbooks, blogs from reputable FODMAP dietitians, or phone apps with up-to-date food lists suggested by credible institutions. Most importantly, avoid monotony by embracing variety with vegetables, grains, and proteins all within portion and ingredient guidelines.

If you are vegetarian, vegan, gluten-free, or have other allergies, carefully cross-reference both safe FODMAP and safe allergen lists before each meal. Focus on legumes with proven low-FODMAP servings (like canned lentils or chickpeas in moderation), tofu, tempeh, and plant-based milks without high-FODMAP additives.

Week one on the Low-FODMAP Elimination Phase is about methodical, all-in commitment. Accuracy in food selection and portion control, vigilance against hidden FODMAPs, and honest, consistent symptom tracking are the tools that transform this challenging week into a period of invaluable learning.

Remember, this isn't about willpower or perfection missteps happen. View any issues as learning opportunities and keep moving forward. In the coming weeks, the process will deepen as you track your progress, introduce variety, and steadily move toward finding your personal balance.

By prioritizing structure, planning, and adaptation, you set yourself up not just for IBS symptom relief, but for an empowered, knowledge-based relationship with food. The elimination phase is temporary, but the groundwork and self-awareness you build in week one will benefit you throughout your IBS management journey.

Week 2 – Deepening Elimination and Symptom Tracking

As you enter week two of the low-FODMAP plan, the focus shifts from initial adjustments to refining your approach: identifying hidden FODMAPs, maintaining balanced nutrition despite restrictions, scrutinizing your food and symptom diaries, tracking bowel habits, and noticing early changes in IBS symptoms.

Addressing Hidden FODMAPs in Processed Foods

Many packaged foods contain concealed FODMAPs. Items that appear compliant often hide high-FODMAP components like garlic, onion, wheat, high fructose corn syrup, chicory root extract (inulin), honey, lactose, or artificial sweeteners (sorbitol, mannitol, xylitol). These occur in products from soups to deli meats, salad dressings, snack bars, and some gluten-free items. Vague label terms such as "natural flavors," "seasonings," or "vegetable powders" can often include FODMAPs unless products are specifically labeled as FODMAP-friendly.

To minimize risk:

- Carefully read all labels, even for familiar brands.
- Choose products labeled low-FODMAP or FODMAP-friendly.
- Avoid foods listing garlic, onion, chicory, inulin, or vague "spices" unless clarified by the manufacturer.
- Watch for sweeteners that end in "-ol."
- Pick simple, whole-food snacks like cucumbers, rice cakes, or homemade popcorn when unsure.

Restaurant and takeout meals also often hide FODMAPs in seasonings, marinades, and sauces, even if labeled gluten-free or digestive-friendly. If uncertain, opt for grilled meats, plain steamed vegetables, and ask for sauces on the side. As you practice, you'll get better at spotting potential FODMAP sources both on labels and menus, lowering the chance of accidental exposure in social or busy settings.

Optimizing Nutrition without Common Culprits

Omitting wheat-based products, dairy, certain fruits, and legumes can make nutritional adequacy a concern, but a well-planned low-FODMAP diet remains balanced and satisfying. There's a wide array of permitted foods: low-FODMAP fruits (strawberries, oranges, blueberries), vegetables (spinach, carrots, eggplant, potatoes, tomatoes), grains (oats, quinoa, rice), and lactose-free dairy or plant-based milk substitutes with no hidden FODMAPs. This range supplies vital nutrients and fiber.

Lean meats, poultry, eggs, firm tofu, and seafood all support protein needs while being naturally low in FODMAPs. Replace wheat with gluten-free grains like quinoa, rice, polenta, or buckwheat. Choose lactose-free or low-lactose dairy options for calcium and probiotics, or fortified plant alternatives.

For healthy fats, use olive oil, low-FODMAP nuts and seeds (walnuts, pecans, chia, pumpkin), and avocado in moderate amounts and note that only up to ⅛ of an avocado is safe per serving.

Planning meals in advance can help sustain both nutrition and adherence:

- ***Example breakfasts***: oats with lactose-free milk, blueberries, and chia seeds.
- ***Example lunches***: grilled chicken with quinoa, roasted carrots, spinach, and olive oil.
- ***Example dinners***: baked salmon with rice, eggplant, and fresh herbs.
- ***Example dnacks***: rice cakes with plain peanut butter (without honey or FODMAP fillers).

Consider keeping a list of favorite low-FODMAP foods and meals handy to combat menu fatigue and inspire variety.

Checklist for Reviewing Food Diaries

Food and symptom diaries are essential for recognizing successful habits and problem areas. A thoughtful review each week helps guide your elimination process and prepares you for reintroduction.

When reviewing:

- Are all foods, drinks, condiments, sauces, gums, and supplements logged?
- Have you included meal and snack times to track possible delayed effects?
- Are serving sizes accurately given, especially for foods with portion limits (avocado, pumpkin seeds)?
- Have any symptoms after meals been noted and related to specific foods?
- Did you record any accidental high-FODMAP exposures, including from restaurants or packaged snacks?
- Are hydration, stress, sleep, and physical activity documented, as these can all affect digestion?

Color coding can help clarify clearly low-FODMAP foods versus questionable ones. Flag processed items for deeper ingredient checks. At week's end, write a short summary: "Three foods I handled well; two moments I risked FODMAP exposure; one improvement for next week."

With time, patterns become clearer such as foods tied to relief or discomfort and these notes can help guide future appointments with healthcare providers.

Guidance on Bowel Habit Monitoring

Since IBS symptoms differ widely, it's critical to monitor not only what you eat, but how your digestion responds. Thorough tracking gives clues to early improvements, pinpoints troubleshooting needs, and separates dietary effects from other influences (like stress or hormones).

Track: Bowel movement frequency and time

- Stool consistency (using something like the Bristol Stool Form Scale).
- Urgency level.
- Pain, bloating, or incomplete emptying.

Also note when bowel movements are normal or comfortable recognizing positive changes reinforces progress and shifts focus from restriction to restored comfort.

Other influences worth recording: sleep, major stress, menstrual cycles, recent illness. For any dramatic or worrying changes (e.g., new severe constipation or diarrhea), consult your healthcare provider.

Many begin to see benefits by week two of reduced bloating or more regular stools though sometimes symptoms persist or temporarily increase as the gut adapts or if there are still hidden FODMAPs. Close monitoring improves your response to changes and outcomes.

Identifying Early Improvements and Challenges

By this stage, consistent elimination and diligent tracking yield insight about your body and the realities of low-FODMAP living. Acknowledging early gains and persistent challenges is crucial for both motivation and planning.

Possible improvements:

- Reduced bloating, pain, or gas.
- More regular or predictable bowel movements.
- Greater confidence with meal prep and eating out thanks to label-reading.
- Enhanced awareness of portions and hidden triggers.

Even slow or partial gains are important, offering real proof that your efforts matter and building motivation. Many find that several small improvements, a little less discomfort, more symptom-free days, or better sleep add up to a meaningful change.

Potential challenges:

- Menu fatigue from limited food variety.

- Social or practical obstacles like office meals, travel, or family gatherings.
- Emotional difficulties, such as frustration over persistent symptoms, food worry, or guilt over mistakes.
- Plateaus in progress, often from ongoing hidden FODMAPs or non-diet factors (stress, sleep issues) interfering with symptom improvement.

Treat these not as failures, but as useful information. Add detail to your food diary, look for new low-FODMAP recipes and foods to vary your menu, and consider professional advice if progress stalls despite your efforts.

Tips for Building Momentum

1. Mark and acknowledge small successes, fewer symptoms and better food identification count as progress.
2. Use a checklist when reviewing diaries and symptoms at week's end to detect both strengths and missed opportunities.
3. Rotate in new low-FODMAP foods and recipes each week to avoid monotony and support diet satisfaction.
4. Share questions or insights with a dietitian, online forum, or trusted person for accountability and support.

By week two's end, your practice in detailed elimination and tracking will set the stage for the next phase: reintroduction. The thoughtful, thorough work you do now will make it much easier to discover your individual food tolerances later.

Remember, the process is not about being perfect but about learning, adapting, and building steady, lasting symptom relief. Each step checking a label, updating your diary, noting a comfort shift is an investment in your long-term gut health and well-being.

Week 3 – Introduction to Systematic Reintroduction

After completing two weeks of strict FODMAP elimination, you are now ready to begin the critical phase of reintroducing FODMAP-containing foods in a controlled, systematic manner. The objective at this stage is not to immediately broaden your diet, but rather to methodically identify which specific FODMAP groups trigger symptoms for you, and which you tolerate well. This knowledge will ultimately empower you to make informed, individualized food choices for the long term, moving toward a more varied and enjoyable eating pattern while managing symptoms of IBS.

Understanding FODMAP Groups and Their Reintroduction

FODMAPs (Fermentable oligosaccharides, disaccharides, monosaccharides, and polyols) are a diverse group of carbohydrates that can cause digestive symptoms in some individuals. The reintroduction phase is designed to test your body's response to each FODMAP subgroup separately:

fructans, lactose, excess fructose, polyols, and galacto-oligosaccharides.

Each of these groups contains unique carbohydrates that may be tolerated differently from one person to another. By isolating each group during testing, you can accurately identify your personal triggers, rather than making broad assumptions about FODMAP sensitivity. This approach minimizes unnecessary dietary restriction and helps you regain dietary diversity where possible.

Step-by-Step Protocol for FODMAP Reintroduction

The systematic reintroduction process involves a structured protocol. Begin by selecting a 'challenge' food that contains only one FODMAP subgroup. For example, choose milk for lactose, wheat bread for fructans, honey for excess fructose, or avocado for polyols. Avoid foods that contain multiple FODMAPs, as these could confound your results and make it difficult to determine which group is responsible for any symptoms.

The recommended protocol is as follows:

1. ***Test one challenge food at a time***: Introduce only one new food per test period, focusing on a single FODMAP group. This isolates the effects and ensures clarity in your results.

2. ***Begin with a small serving***: On Day 1, start with a conservative portion typically an amount you might eat in one meal. This reduces the risk of triggering severe symptoms and provides a gentle test for tolerance.
3. ***Gradually increase the portion***: If you experience no symptoms after the initial serving, try a slightly larger portion on Day 2, and again on Day 3 if the previous days were symptom-free. This stepwise approach helps establish the upper limit of your tolerance for each FODMAP group.
4. ***Return to the elimination baseline between challenges***: After completing a three-day trial with a challenge food, revert to your strict low-FODMAP baseline diet for at least two days. This 'washout' period ensures any lingering effects of the previous challenge subside before you move on to the next FODMAP group.
5. ***Maintain a clear schedule***: Repeat this process for each FODMAP group, always allowing for a washout period and documenting each step carefully.

Managing Timing and Spacing of Food Challenges

Spacing out your food challenges is essential for accurate results. Always allow at least two symptom-free washout days between challenge foods. This prevents overlap in digestive responses and ensures that any symptoms can be confidently attributed to the food you are currently testing.

If you do experience symptoms, stop the reintroduction immediately, return to the strict elimination diet, and wait until you are symptom-free before proceeding. This patience is crucial for accurately identifying which FODMAPs are problematic for you, and for preventing unnecessary discomfort or confusion.

Detailed Record-Keeping: The Key to Reliable Results

Meticulous documentation is a cornerstone of the reintroduction phase. Each day, record the following:

- The specific food and the portion size you consumed
- The exact time of consumption
- Any digestive symptoms (such as bloating, abdominal pain, gas, or diarrhea)
- Any extra-digestive symptoms (such as fatigue, headaches, or mood changes)
- The time of onset and the severity of any symptoms

Comprehensive logs help distinguish real FODMAP sensitivities from unrelated discomforts. Consistency is vital; use a standardized diary or symptom chart to ensure accuracy. Additionally, make note of external factors that could influence your symptoms, such as emotional stress, lack of sleep, physical activity, or concurrent illness. Such factors can confound your results if not considered.

A sample entry in your food and symptom diary might look like this:

- ***Date***: Monday, Week 3, Day 1
- ***Challenge food***: Wheat bread (fructans), 1 slice
- ***Time consumed***: 8:00 am
- ***Symptoms***: Mild bloating at 11:00 am, resolved by 1:00 pm
- ***External factors***: Slept poorly the previous night

By tracking these details for each challenge, you create a reliable record that will allow you and your healthcare provider to make informed decisions about your diet going forward.

Responding to Symptoms During Reintroduction

If you notice any symptoms during a food challenge, take note of the type, timing, and severity. Common symptoms include abdominal pain, bloating, changes in bowel habits, or other digestive discomfort. If symptoms are mild, you may choose to continue the challenge with caution; however, if symptoms are moderate to severe, discontinue the current food and return to the elimination phase. Wait until you are symptom-free for at least 48 hours before attempting a new challenge. This ensures that your results are not muddled by lingering effects from a previous reaction.

Building Your Diet After FODMAP Reintroduction

Once you have systematically worked through each FODMAP group and identified which subgroups and foods are well-tolerated, you can begin to craft a personalized, less restrictive diet. The goal is to reintroduce as many foods as possible without triggering symptoms, improving both the nutritional adequacy and enjoyment of your meals.

Begin by incorporating well-tolerated foods from your challenge phase into balanced meals. Combine these with proteins and vegetables that you have continued to tolerate during the elimination phase. For example, you might enjoy grilled chicken or fish paired with low-FODMAP vegetables such as zucchini, carrots, or spinach, and a moderate serving of a FODMAP-tested food, like a slice of sourdough bread if you have tolerated wheat-based fructans.

If you have successfully reintroduced lactose, you can enjoy dairy products such as lactose-free milk or yogurt. If both fructans and lactose are tolerated, a breakfast of oats with milk and banana slices becomes an option.

Here are a few meal ideas that reflect successful FODMAP reintroduction:

- Grilled chicken breast with sautéed zucchini and carrots, served with sourdough bread (if wheat-based fructans are tolerated)

- Baked salmon with a side of quinoa and steamed green beans, topped with a drizzle of olive oil
- Oats prepared with lactose-free milk, topped with banana slices or blueberries, as tolerated
- Stir-fried tofu with bell peppers and rice, seasoned with garlic-infused oil (garlic flavor without the FODMAP content)

As you expand your diet, continue to monitor your symptoms and update your food and symptom diary. Flexibility is important if you find that a food you once tolerated begins to provoke symptoms, consider pausing its consumption and retesting at a later date. Likewise, some foods may become more tolerable over time as your gut adapts or your overall health improves.

Consulting with a registered dietitian experienced in the low-FODMAP protocol can be invaluable during this process. A dietitian can help interpret your records, troubleshoot challenges, and ensure your diet remains balanced and nutritionally adequate as you expand your food choices.

The reintroduction phase of the low-FODMAP diet is as much an exercise in self-discovery as it is a clinical process. By patiently, systematically testing each FODMAP group and documenting your experiences, you lay the foundation for a diet that meets both your nutritional needs and your personal preferences. The ultimate goal is not perpetual restriction, but a flexible, enjoyable, and sustainable way of eating that supports your digestive health and overall well-being.

Week 4 – Building Your Personal Low-FODMAP Blueprint

After three weeks of strict elimination and careful reintroduction, you've arrived at a pivotal point in your low-FODMAP journey. Week 4 is not just about following rules but about actively integrating everything you've learned to create a dietary blueprint tailored to your unique needs.

By charting your personal FODMAP tolerances, you can enjoy greater dietary freedom while consistently managing your IBS symptoms. This chapter will guide you in solidifying your newfound insights, avoiding unnecessary long-term restrictions, planning balanced meals, adapting portion sizes for relief, and smoothly transitioning your diet for various real-world scenarios.

Charting Individual FODMAP Tolerances

The primary goal of week 4 is to translate your symptom observations from the reintroduction phase into clear, actionable guidance for your daily eating. Begin by reviewing your food and symptom diary, focusing on your body's responses to each FODMAP subgroup. Note which foods and categories triggered symptoms and at what quantities, as well as those you tolerated without issue.

To chart your individual FODMAP tolerances, try the following steps:

- Create a list or table, grouping foods by their FODMAP category (such as fructans, lactose, excess fructose, and polyols).
- For each category, identify test foods from your reintroduction phase and rate your tolerance: well tolerated, moderate symptoms, or clear trigger.
- Record specific portion sizes that were tolerated, as FODMAP sensitivity is often dose-dependent.
- Where necessary, highlight foods that are borderline and may require further testing down the line.

Charting in this way helps transform your raw experience into a living resource, which you can update over time as you refine your food choices and challenge new foods. This personalized list will not only guide you now but also become a valuable reference when navigating meals, social occasions, or product labels in the future.

Strategies to Avoid Unnecessary Long-Term Restriction

After several weeks of eliminating high-FODMAP foods, it can feel safer to keep your diet very restricted, especially if you've finally found some symptom relief. However, unnecessarily long-term restriction may prevent you from enjoying a varied, satisfying diet and could risk nutrient inadequacies or social limitations. The key is to reintroduce as much dietary variety as your symptoms allow and to avoid restricting foods you can tolerate.

Here are evidence-based strategies to avoid getting "stuck" in the elimination phase:

1. Only permanently avoid foods or FODMAP groups that clearly and consistently trigger symptoms. If a food causes occasional, mild issues, consider retesting in the future at different portion sizes or as part of mixed meals.
2. For foods you tolerate, even if only in small amounts, try gradually increasing your serving sizes over time to test your threshold. Intolerance often depends on the dose; many people handle moderate amounts, particularly when foods are combined in mixed meals rather than eaten alone.
3. Rotate tolerated foods from all major food groups to ensure a balanced intake of nutrients.

4. Use your symptom-free foods to maintain dietary variety. This flexibility is not only protective against boredom but supports gut health through exposure to a diverse range of fibers and micronutrients.
5. Remember that your tolerances are dynamic; stress, illness, or medications can temporarily alter your digestive sensitivity, so be open to periodic retesting.

The takeaway is to use your personalized list to expand your food choices as much as possible while managing IBS symptoms striking a healthy balance between comfort and quality of life.

Guidelines for Balanced and Flexible Meal Planning

Planning satisfying and balanced meals is essential for both symptom management and overall health. Many traditional meal plans become monotonous or nutritionally incomplete during the low-FODMAP process, but with careful structure and creativity, you can achieve variety while respecting your personal tolerances.

Here are practical meal planning guidelines to follow:

1. Aim for a mix of lean proteins, healthy fats, low-FODMAP grains and starches, and a variety of tolerated fruits and vegetables in every meal.

2. Use your "tolerated" FODMAP foods to add diversity, color, and flavor. For example, if you discover you are not sensitive to a particular polyol, include small portions of that fruit or vegetable throughout the week.
3. Plan your meals on a weekly basis, incorporating at least one new or previously restricted food each week for ongoing variety and challenge, as appropriate.
4. Include low-FODMAP dairy or lactose-free alternatives to ensure calcium and vitamin D intake, unless you tolerate small amounts of lactose.
5. Choose high-fiber options from your "safe" list such as oats, chia seeds, or low-FODMAP vegetables to support digestive regularity and the health of your gut microbiome.
6. When adapted recipes are needed, leverage resources that specify swaps and substitutions suitable for your tolerances; many low-FODMAP recipe collections also integrate these practices, ensuring both nutritional adequacy and taste variety.

A weekly meal plan that pools the foods you tolerate and adapts recipes as necessary helps guard against nutritional gaps and mealtime monotony. Being proactive rather than reactive ensures you're less likely to default to restrictive habits or get caught off guard by unplanned meals.

Adapting Portion Sizes for Sustained Symptom Relief

FODMAP tolerance is not always all-or-nothing; most people have a symptom threshold that depends on both quantity and frequency of exposure. Even when you've identified trigger foods, you may be able to enjoy them in smaller quantities without adverse effects.

To adapt portion sizes for long-term comfort, follow these practical steps:

1. Learn your personal portion thresholds by referring to your week 3 diary the amount and frequency at which symptoms appeared are valuable clues.
2. For foods you tolerate at small amounts, plan to include them in moderation, spreading intake throughout the week instead of all at once.
3. Be mindful of cumulative FODMAP load within a single meal; several moderate-FODMAP foods together may exceed your individual tolerance, even if each would be tolerated alone.
4. Track any symptoms that arise if you intentionally increase a portion, and adjust downward if needed. Regular, honest feedback is key to finding lasting comfort and flexibility.
5. If eating out or during travel, err on the side of caution with known limit foods, but don't avoid them entirely unless you are certain they are problematic at all doses.

Sustained symptom control comes from matching your unique sensitivities identified through systematic reintroduction to realistic, enjoyable portion sizes. Over time, you may notice your ability to tolerate certain foods grows, especially as your gut adjusts and adapts, so periodic retesting is wise.

Dietary Transition Tips for Social and Travel Contexts

One of the greatest challenges on a low-FODMAP plan is maintaining your progress outside the comfort of your home kitchen. Social gatherings, restaurants, and travel can raise anxiety about hidden FODMAPs, cross-contact, or unpredictable meal content. With a strategic approach, you can minimize stress, maintain symptom control, and still embrace the experiences that matter to you.

Consider these actionable strategies for dining out and traveling:

1. Plan ahead by researching restaurants or menus whenever possible. Many eateries now accommodate dietary requests, and low-FODMAP-friendly dishes are increasingly available.
2. For social events, don't hesitate to communicate your needs to hosts. Offer to bring a dish you know you tolerate, ensuring you have at least one safe option.

3. Carry portable "safe foods" for travel such as gluten-free crackers, small packets of nut butter (if tolerated), firm bananas, rice cakes, or lactose-free snack packs. Having these on hand helps avoid risky impulsive choices.
4. Learn basic keywords for FODMAP triggers in other languages if traveling abroad, or keep a printed card explaining your needs for non-English-speaking staff.
5. Prioritize portion control when you cannot be sure of full ingredient lists. Sticking to small servings and mixing foods with known tolerances reduces the risk of symptoms from hidden FODMAPs.
6. When uncertain about a dish, ask questions about preparation methods; for instance, requesting salad dressings or sauces on the side often grants more control.
7. Be patient with yourself if symptoms occur, return to your safe foods temporarily, and resume your established plan as conditions allow.

Travel and social situations are opportunities to actively use your personalized blueprint, rather than reasons to abandon it. Over time, your growing confidence and resourcefulness guided by your personal FODMAP chart and flexible meal plans will transform these scenarios from obstacles into experiences you can embrace and enjoy.

Week 4 marks your transition from following "the low-FODMAP diet" to living out your own version of a highly individualized, sustainable approach that prioritizes symptom control, dietary satisfaction, and flexibility. This is not a static endpoint, but the beginning of an ongoing process. Your personal IBS management will evolve as your tolerances, lifestyle, and food environment change.

Use your individual FODMAP tolerance chart as your primary compass for food choices, always aiming to maximize dietary variety and enjoyment. Avoid unnecessary restriction by periodically challenging former trigger foods, especially if your health circumstances or stress levels shift. Plan balanced, colorful meals designed around foods that support both your health and your happiness, and adapt portion sizes based on feedback from your gut.

Develop practical routines for socializing and traveling that align with your blueprint, and remember: slip-ups are part of the journey, not signs of failure. With each week, your knowledge and confidence grow, bringing you closer to a richer, more predictable life with IBS.

Your personal low-FODMAP blueprint, a document that began as a symptom diary is now a practical manual, ready to guide you through daily decisions, novel experiences, and every meal in between. This living plan will ensure that you, not your symptoms, are in charge of what, how, and where you eat.

In the next chapter, you'll find a range of practical recipes, snack ideas, and customizable planning tools all designed to help you sustain your progress and keep your blueprint fresh and enjoyable long after these initial four weeks are done.

Recipes and Practical Planning Tools

Making the low-FODMAP diet sustainable requires more than knowing ingredients—it calls for adaptable recipes, snack and beverage ideas, and planning strategies that fit your daily life. In this chapter, you'll find foundational recipes for all meals, guidance on customizing recipes for allergens, visual serving size aids, and step-by-step planning templates. These tools help translate knowledge into confident, enjoyable everyday eating.

Core Low-FODMAP Recipes for Each Meal

A reliable set of low-FODMAP recipes prepares you for any meal, whether at home or on-the-go. Below are simple, flexible recipes for breakfast, lunch, dinner, and dessert, all easy to batch-cook and customize.

Breakfast

Oatmeal with Berries and Chia

Ingredients:

- 1/2 cup gluten-free rolled oats
- 1 cup water or lactose-free milk
- 1/4 cup strawberries, sliced
- 1/4 cup blueberries
- 1/4 cup raspberries (optional)
- 1 tablespoon chia seeds
- 1 tablespoon maple syrup (optional)

Instructions:

1. In a small saucepan, combine the oats and water or lactose-free milk. Bring to a gentle boil over medium heat.
2. Reduce heat to low and simmer, stirring occasionally, for 5-7 minutes or until the oats are soft and have absorbed most of the liquid.
3. Remove from heat. Spoon the oatmeal into a bowl.
4. Top with strawberries, blueberries, raspberries (if using), and chia seeds.
5. Drizzle with maple syrup if desired. Serve warm. This recipe can be made ahead and reheated for a quick breakfast.

Low-FODMAP Frittata Muffins

Ingredients:

- 6 large eggs
- 1 cup fresh spinach, chopped
- 1/2 cup red bell pepper, diced
- 1/4 cup feta cheese, crumbled (use a hard feta for lower lactose)
- 1/4 teaspoon salt
- 1/4 teaspoon black pepper
- Nonstick cooking spray or muffin liners

Instructions:

1. Preheat your oven to 350°F (175°C). Lightly grease a 6-cup muffin tin with nonstick spray or use muffin liners.
2. In a medium bowl, beat the eggs. Stir in the chopped spinach, diced red bell pepper, crumbled feta, salt, and pepper.
3. Divide the egg mixture evenly among the 6 muffin cups.
4. Bake for 18-22 minutes, or until the muffins are set and lightly golden.
5. Let cool slightly before removing from the tin. Enjoy warm, or let cool completely and store in the refrigerator for up to 4 days. These are perfect for grab-and-go mornings.

Lunch

Quinoa Veggie Bowl

Ingredients:

- 1 cup cooked quinoa
- 1 cup fresh spinach leaves
- 1/2 cup shredded carrots
- 1/2 cup cherry tomatoes, halved
- 1 grilled chicken breast (sliced) or 1/2 cup firm tofu (cubed), if tolerated
- 1 tablespoon olive oil
- 1 tablespoon fresh lemon juice
- Salt and pepper, to taste

Instructions:

1. In a large bowl, combine the cooked quinoa, spinach, carrots, and cherry tomatoes.
2. Add the grilled chicken breast slices or, if preferred and tolerated, the cubed firm tofu.
3. Drizzle olive oil and lemon juice over the mixture.
4. Season with salt and pepper to taste.
5. Toss gently to combine all ingredients. Swap out any vegetables as needed according to dietary preferences or tolerances. Monitor portions if required.

Grilled Chicken Salad

Ingredients:

- 2 cups mixed salad greens
- 1/2 cucumber, sliced
- 1/2 cup roasted pumpkin cubes
- 1 grilled chicken breast, sliced
- 2 tablespoons sunflower seeds
- 1 tablespoon olive oil
- 1 teaspoon mustard
- 1 tablespoon fresh lemon juice
- Salt and pepper, to taste
- Vegetarian Option: Substitute chicken with 1/2 cup cooked chickpeas, only if personally tolerated after reintroduction.

Instructions:

1. In a large salad bowl, combine mixed greens, cucumber, and roasted pumpkin.
2. Add the grilled chicken slices. For a vegetarian option, substitute chicken with cooked chickpeas if tolerated.
3. Sprinkle sunflower seeds over the top.
4. In a small bowl, whisk together olive oil, mustard, lemon juice, salt, and pepper to make the dressing.
5. Drizzle the dressing over the salad and toss gently to combine.
6. Serve immediately.

Dinner

Low-FODMAP Stir-Fry

Ingredients:

- 1 lb beef, chicken breast, or tempeh, cut into strips
- 1 cup carrots, julienned
- 1 cup zucchini, sliced into half-moons
- 1 cup bell pepper, sliced
- 1 cup bean sprouts
- 2 tablespoons garlic-infused olive oil (ensure garlic solids are removed)
- 2 tablespoons gluten-free tamari (soy sauce)
- Steamed rice or rice noodles, to serve
- Salt and pepper to taste

Instructions:

1. Heat the garlic-infused olive oil in a large skillet or wok over medium-high heat. Make sure to use only the infused oil and discard any garlic pieces.
2. Add the beef, chicken, or tempeh strips and sauté for 3-4 minutes until browned and cooked through. Remove from the pan and set aside.
3. Add carrots, zucchini, and bell pepper to the skillet. Stir-fry for 3-4 minutes until just tender.

4. Return the cooked protein to the pan, add bean sprouts, and stir in the gluten-free tamari. Cook for another 1-2 minutes until everything is heated through.
5. Season with salt and pepper to taste. Serve over steamed rice or rice noodles.

Baked Salmon with Roasted Veggies

Ingredients:

- 2 salmon fillets (about 6 oz each)
- 1 cup carrots, cut into sticks
- 1 cup parsnip, cut into sticks
- 1 cup green beans, trimmed
- 2 tablespoons olive oil
- 1 teaspoon dried or fresh dill
- Salt and pepper to taste
- 1 cup baby potatoes, boiled

Instructions:

1. Preheat your oven to 400°F (200°C).
2. Place the carrots, parsnip, and green beans on a baking sheet. Drizzle with 1 tablespoon of olive oil, season with salt and pepper, and toss to coat.
3. Push the vegetables to the sides of the baking sheet and place the salmon fillets in the center. Drizzle salmon with the remaining olive oil and sprinkle with dill, salt, and pepper.
4. Bake for 15-18 minutes, or until the salmon is cooked through and the vegetables are tender.

5. While the salmon and veggies are baking, boil the baby potatoes in salted water until fork-tender, about 12-15 minutes. Drain.
6. Serve the baked salmon and roasted veggies with a side of boiled potatoes for a complete meal.

Dessert

Low-FODMAP Fruit Parfait

Ingredients:

- 1 cup lactose-free yogurt
- 1/3 cup fresh strawberries, hulled and sliced
- 1 small kiwi, peeled and sliced
- 1/4 cup gluten-free granola (ensure it does not contain high-FODMAP ingredients)

Instructions:

1. Spoon half of the lactose-free yogurt into the bottom of a glass or bowl.
2. Add half of the sliced strawberries and kiwi on top of the yogurt layer.
3. Sprinkle half of the gluten-free granola over the fruit.
4. Repeat the layers with the remaining yogurt, fruit, and granola.
5. Serve immediately, or cover and refrigerate for up to a few hours.

Tips:

- Avoid using dried fruits or adding extra sweeteners to keep the parfait low in FODMAPs.
- For added flavor, top with a few fresh mint leaves if desired.

Feel free to adapt these core recipes based on your personal tolerances. As you reintroduce foods, gradually incorporate new ingredients to expand your menu.

Snack and Beverage Suggestions

Strategic snacking helps maintain energy and avoid digestive discomfort. Select snacks and drinks that are quick, satisfying, and safe for your gut.

Snack Ideas

- Rice cakes with natural peanut butter (peanuts and salt only)
- Firm cheese slices and cucumber rounds
- Low-FODMAP trail mix: pumpkin seeds, sunflower seeds, puffed rice, and a few dried cranberries (use sparingly)
- Carrot and bell pepper sticks with a dip of lactose-free yogurt, lemon, and herbs
- Hard-boiled eggs for portable protein
- Air-popped plain popcorn with olive oil or sea salt

Beverage Ideas

- Water infused with orange, lemon, or cucumber slices
- Peppermint or ginger tea for digestive support
- Lactose-free milk or rice, oat, or almond milk (check for high-FODMAP additives)
- Plain green or black tea
- Small smoothies using allowed fruits such as spinach, cucumber, and pineapple blended with lactose-free yogurt

These options deliver flavor and nourishment without compromising low-FODMAP goals.

Adapting Recipes for Common Allergens

Many with IBS have other food allergies. The following substitutions help you adapt recipes for gluten, dairy, nut, or egg restrictions, while keeping FODMAPs low.

1. ***Gluten-Free***: Low-FODMAP eating already excludes most high-gluten grains, but always choose certified gluten-free oats, pastas, and breads to avoid traces. For baking, try rice, potato, or quinoa flour.
2. ***Dairy-Free***: Use lactose-free milk or plant-based milks (oat, almond, rice—avoid those with chicory or inulin). Coconut or lactose-free yogurt is preferred for dairy-free needs. Omit cheese or swap for nutritional yeast as a savory flavor replacement.

3. ***Nut-Free***: Omit nuts from recipes; replace with seeds like pumpkin or sunflower for crunch and nutrients.
4. ***Egg-Free***: For baking, use a "chia or flax egg" (1 tbsp ground chia or flaxseed with 3 tbsp water, set to thicken). Use tofu scramble in place of eggs for breakfast, if soy is tolerated.

Check ingredient labels and adapt recipe amounts as needed to maintain both safety and taste.

Portion Control Visual Aids and Serving Size Charts

Serving size is crucial: even low-FODMAP foods can be problematic in excess. Visual guides make portioning intuitive and help prevent symptoms.

Portion Visuals

- ***Protein***: Palm of your hand (about 3–4 ounces cooked)
- ***Grains***: One cupped hand (about ½ cup cooked)
- ***Vegetables***: Two open hands or a heaped fist per meal
- ***Fruit***: Tennis ball-sized or one handful

Table 1: Serving Size Chart

Food Group	Example Foods	Safe Portion (per meal)
Grains	Rice, quinoa, gluten-free oats	½ cup cooked
Protein	Chicken, eggs, firm tofu	3-4 oz (palm-sized portion)
Vegetables	Carrots, zucchini, spinach	½-1 cup cooked or 1-2 cups raw

Fruit	Strawberries, kiwi, oranges	1 medium fruit or ½ cup sliced
Dairy (lactose-free)	Milk, yogurt	Up to 1 cup
Nuts & Seeds	Sunflower, pumpkin, chia	1–2 tbsp
Fats	Olive oil, butter	1 tbsp

These guidelines support appropriate intake and make reading package labels easier. Adjust portions based on your individual tolerance, and track responses in your diary.

Weekly Meal Prep and Planning Tools

Planning reduces stress, prevents accidental FODMAP overexposure, and streamlines your routine. A weekly meal planner and categorized shopping list keep your meals varied and help manage your time and food budget.

Sample Meal Planner

1. Pick 2–3 breakfast options (e.g., overnight oats, frittata muffins).
2. Select 3–4 lunch ideas (quinoa veggie bowl, chicken salad), use leftovers for efficiency.
3. Choose 4–5 dinners (baked salmon, stir-fry, brown rice pilaf, grilled fish).
4. Batch-cook once or twice a week.
5. List preferred snacks and beverages to avoid last-minute high-FODMAP temptations.
6. Make a shopping list broken down by food category.

Table 2: Sample Weekly Layout

Day	Breakfast	Lunch	Dinner	Snacks
Mon	Overnight oats	Quinoa veggie bowl	Salmon with roasted veggies	Rice cakes, fruit, yogurt
Tue	Frittata muffins	Chicken salad	Stir-fry with noodles	Popcorn, cheese, cucumber slices
Wed	Overnight oats	Leftover stir-fry	Brown rice pilaf with tofu	Trail mix, carrot sticks
Thu				
Fri				

Shopping List Template

- ***Proteins***: Chicken breast, tofu, eggs, salmon
- ***Grains***: Gluten-free oats, brown rice, rice noodles
- ***Vegetables***: Spinach, carrots, zucchini, green beans, salad greens
- ***Dairy alternatives***: Lactose-free yogurt, plant-based milk
- ***Fruits***: Strawberries, blueberries, kiwi
- ***Pantry***: Olive oil, sunflower seeds
- ***Snacks***: Rice cakes, popcorn kernels

Keep staples on hand, check what you already own to reduce kitchen waste, and update your list as preferences change.

Batch Cooking and Prep Tips

1. Wash and chop vegetables ahead; store in airtight containers.
2. Cook grains in bulk and refrigerate portions for the week.
3. Prepare extra protein (like chicken or hard-boiled eggs) to speed up meals.
4. Label leftovers with dates to avoid spoilage.

Advanced Planning Tactics

- For families with varied needs, color-code meal plans per person. Tech-savvy users may benefit from meal-planning apps that also organize grocery lists.
- Organization builds routine while still allowing flexibility. A set plan helps avoid moments of hunger panic and ensures you always have something safe and satisfying ready.

Turning Plans into Practice

With these recipes, portion tools, and planning templates, the low-FODMAP diet becomes empowering instead of restrictive. Batch-cooking, adapting for allergens, or having trusted snacks on hand transforms FODMAP management into a practical lifestyle.

Continue to use a food and symptom diary to personalize your plan and adjust as needed. Review and update your meal planner regularly based on what you enjoy and how your gut responds—consistency and adaptability are both key. With planning and creativity, managing IBS with a low-FODMAP approach becomes not just achievable, but genuinely pleasant.

Troubleshooting, Long-term Maintenance, and Professional Support

Managing IBS with a low-FODMAP diet doesn't end once you identify trigger foods or complete the initial protocol. True long-term success requires troubleshooting ongoing symptoms, maintaining nutrition, adapting to new life situations, and knowing when to seek professional help. This chapter explains core strategies for addressing hurdles, preserving your well-being, and keeping up with research as recommendations change.

Solutions for Persistent Symptoms During the Diet

Even when following the diet closely, IBS symptoms can linger or return. Use the following steps to address persistent issues:

1. ***Re-examine Food Choices***: Hidden FODMAPs lurk in packaged and homemade foods. Check labels and recipes for ingredients like high-fructose corn syrup,

honey, inulin, or wheat-based thickeners. Don't overlook additives in spices, sauces, and non-dairy milks, which often carry unexpected FODMAPs.

2. ***Confirm Portion Control***: Tolerance to FODMAPs depends on the amount: even allowed foods can trigger symptoms if eaten in excess. For example, a small slice of avocado is fine, but a larger portion isn't. Compare your servings to recommended amounts, downsize portions, and keep meals simple as you reassess.
3. ***Audit for Cross-Contamination***: Symptoms may persist because high-FODMAP foods contaminate shared prep areas or utensils. If you share a kitchen or eat out, explain your needs clearly and ask for separate food preparation to minimize risk.
4. ***Consider Other Triggers***: IBS is affected by more than FODMAPs: high-fat foods, caffeine, alcohol, and spicy ingredients often cause problems too. Stress or lack of sleep can also worsen symptoms. Monitor your entire lifestyle, not just diet.
5. ***Try a Basic Meal Reset***: If nothing helps, eat a few days of simple, well-tolerated foods like plain proteins, white rice, carrots, and allowed oils. Observe symptoms, then gradually reintroduce foods one at a time to isolate any offenders. This "reset" helps clarify what's causing trouble.

6. ***Seek New Recipes to Prevent Monotony***: Boredom can make it harder to stick to your plan. Find new low-FODMAP recipes for snacks, meals, or desserts to keep your diet appealing and limit the urge to "cheat".

Criteria for Seeking Medical or Dietitian Advice

While many navigate the low-FODMAP process alone, some situations need professional input:

1. **Persistent or Worsening Symptoms**

   If careful elimination hasn't relieved symptoms, consult a doctor or registered dietitian. Ongoing trouble can indicate another issue, such as celiac disease, inflammatory bowel disease, or infection—conditions needing medical intervention.

2. **Significant Weight Loss, Deficiencies, or New Symptoms**

   Unplanned weight loss, fatigue, skin changes, or fresh digestive complaints may signal nutritional problems. A dietitian can review your intake and rebalance your plan without triggering IBS.

3. **Difficulty with Compliance or Meal Planning**

   If low-FODMAP meal prep or shopping feels too difficult, a dietitian with FODMAP experience can supply tailored, practical support, helping you avoid common errors.

4. **Coexisting Allergies or Health Conditions**

   Managing additional restrictions lactose intolerance, nut allergies, diabetes makes dietary planning complex and raises the risk of deficiencies. A dietitian ensures your nutrition and safety aren't compromised.

5. **Emotional or Psychological Stress**

   If IBS or dietary changes cause anxiety, persistent food fears, or social withdrawal, seek help from a dietitian and, if needed, a mental health professional.

Maintaining Nutritional Adequacy Long-Term

Sticking to low FODMAPs for extended periods can create nutritional gaps, particularly if you haven't completed reintroduction or are avoiding many foods. To prevent deficiencies:

1. ***Finish the Reintroduction Phase***: The diet's goal is to pinpoint triggers, not exclude all FODMAPs long term. Skipping reintroduction narrows your diet and can cut key nutrients. Test each FODMAP group systematically, note your responses, and restore tolerated foods for variety and nutrition.

2. ***Monitor Dietary Variety***: Eat a wide range of naturally low-FODMAP proteins, produce, grains, and healthy fats. Rotate your foods frequently to boost nutrient diversity and benefit gut bacteria.
3. ***Use Supplements Only as Needed***: If you avoid animal proteins or fortified grains, certain nutrients (calcium, vitamin D, B-vitamins, iron) may require supplementation. Always check with a healthcare provider before starting, as some supplements contain high-FODMAP fillers.
4. ***Practice Balanced, Adaptable Meal Planning***: Use reliable meal plans emphasizing whole foods and simplicity. Meals should mix lean proteins (eggs, fish, tofu), safe carbs (potatoes, quinoa), and a range of low-FODMAP fiber sources like greens, zucchini, or berries.
5. ***Keep a Food and Symptom Diary***: Even after progress, occasional symptoms and food tracking helps spot patterns before deficiencies or issues arise.

Adapting Your Plan as Life Changes

Long-term success requires flexibility as situations evolve new jobs, travel, or changing routines. Strategies for smooth adaptation include:

1. ***Plan for Busy Times***: Prepping meals in advance on weekends, in batches, or as freezer portions saves time

when life is hectic. Keep shelf-stable options (canned tuna, rice cakes, lactose-free milk) for convenience.

2. ***Eating Out and Social Events***: State your needs confidently; check menus in advance and call restaurants when necessary. Order simply prepared items, like grilled meats or plain salads.
3. ***Travel Solutions***: Bring safe snacks (boiled eggs, small bananas, oranges, cereal packs) and check for grocery stores or kitchen access at your destination.
4. ***Coordinating with Other Health Goals***: If you're working toward weight loss, muscle gain, or athletic milestones, balance macronutrients within FODMAP limits. A dietitian can help you meet these needs using appropriate carbs, fats, and meal timing.
5. ***Re-evaluate FODMAP Tolerances***: Sensitivity to FODMAPs may change with age, health status, or lifestyle. Every six to twelve months, retest individual FODMAP groups to keep your diet responsive and relevant.
6. ***Supporting Non-FODMAP Households***: If family members eat differently, designate FODMAP-safe storage and prep areas. Plan flexible meals like taco bars or salads that each person can customize.

Adapting your plan as life changes helps ensure long-term success and minimizes stress. Staying proactive and responsive to your needs allows you to maintain a healthy and enjoyable diet, no matter what life brings.

Staying Informed on IBS and FODMAP Developments

Research in nutrition and gut health is always evolving. Keeping up will help your approach remain effective:

1. ***Rely on Reputable Sources***: Use well-established research groups, academic institutions, and advocacy organizations for updates about guidelines, food lists, and new therapies.
2. ***Watch for Updates in Food Status and Portions***: Testing sometimes reclassifies foods as high or low FODMAP, or changes advised portion sizes. Check lists regularly to discover new options or updated recommendations.
3. ***Attend Educational Events***: Look for workshops or webinars from nutritionists, hospitals, or patient organizations. These offer Q&A and connections with experts or peers.
4. ***Use Reliable Apps and Digital Tools***: Quality mobile apps from official sources often update food databases and aid in tracking foods and symptoms. These are especially handy when traveling or trying new foods.
5. ***Annual Check-ins with Your Dietitian***: As research progresses, your care team might offer updated reintroductions, probiotic guidance, or fiber adjustments. Annual reviews keep your plan current and evidence-based.

Staying current with IBS and FODMAP research ensures your dietary approach remains both safe and effective. Regularly updating your knowledge empowers you to make informed decisions for better gut health.

Practical Example: Overcoming a Holiday Setback

Suppose months of symptom control are undone during a holiday by bloating and pain. Here's what you do:

1. Review food diaries for hidden triggers, like desserts or sauces.
2. Return to simple, safe meals for several days and track improvements.
3. If symptoms persist, see a professional to reassess or address other causes.
4. Seek new low-FODMAP recipes for future festive meals to keep the experience positive.

These steps help turn setbacks into opportunities to reinforce your knowledge and practices.

Effective, sustained relief from IBS symptoms with a low-FODMAP diet relies on systematic troubleshooting, ongoing nutritional vigilance, adaptation to life changes, and knowing when to seek expert support. By focusing on steady dietary balance, staying alert to new findings, and ensuring your approach fits your evolving needs, you can transform the diet from a short-term fix into an enduring, empowering routine.

Conclusion

As you reach the end of your four-week low-FODMAP journey, it's important to take a moment to reflect on your accomplishments, new insights, and the foundation you've built for lasting IBS relief. This structured process has equipped you with practical skills, a deeper understanding, and a personalized route to better digestive health. The path doesn't end here; it simply marks the beginning of ongoing self-care and adaptation tailored to your unique needs.

Throughout these weeks, you've learned how to systematically remove foods high in FODMAPs and gradually test your individual tolerance to specific ingredients. By relying on meal planning tools, food symptom diaries, and a roster of satisfying low-FODMAP recipes, you've experienced how a mindful approach can help identify your trigger foods and reduce debilitating symptoms.. Seeing symptom patterns shift sometimes even before the end of the first week—reinforces the potential for meaningful change and enhanced day-to-day comfort.

Equally important, you've collected valuable data about your personal tolerance, allowing you to build a sustainable eating plan that balances variety with gut-friendly choices. By the fourth week, most participants are able to define their safe foods, identify flexible meal options, and gain confidence in their dietary decisions. This process doesn't just clarify what to avoid; it offers clear guidance on what you can happily enjoy while reducing the risk of unnecessary restrictions that could impact nutrition and quality of life.

Sustaining your progress means embracing continuous self-monitoring. IBS is known to fluctuate over time, influenced by stress, travel, social events, and unforeseen dietary exposures. Make it a habit to revisit your food-symptom diary when symptoms arise, review product ingredient lists for hidden FODMAPs, and monitor shifts in bowel habits as your routine or environment changes. Should new symptoms emerge, methodically assessing recent meals and contextual factors can help you adjust quickly and with confidence.

Adaptability is key as life evolves. You might face new challenges such as dining out, holidays, or changes in living situation. Lean on the practical planning strategies you've learned: refer to familiar recipes, use your meal planner template, and practice open communication with hosts, friends, or restaurant staff about your needs. Flexibility allows you to protect your gut health without feeling confined or deprived.

Crucially, do not hesitate to seek support on your ongoing journey. The expertise of registered dietitians, GI specialists, or therapists with experience in digestive health can be invaluable for troubleshooting, ensuring balanced nutrition, and guiding further reintroduction if your symptom patterns change. Connecting with others who are also managing IBS—through support groups or online communities can offer encouragement, troubleshooting tips, and a much-needed sense of belonging when facing setbacks or uncertainty.

Remember, your commitment over these four weeks demonstrates that change is possible, and that your efforts pay real dividends in well-being and self-empowerment. Use the knowledge, confidence, and community resources you've gained to maintain the positive momentum. Sustaining IBS relief is an ongoing process of self-awareness, flexibility, and seeking guidance when needed, one that you are now exceptionally well-prepared to continue.

FAQS

Are the Low-FODMAP and gluten-free diets the same?

No, though often confused, the low-FODMAP and gluten-free diets serve different purposes. The low-FODMAP diet manages irritable bowel syndrome (IBS) by restricting certain carbohydrates that can trigger symptoms like bloating, pain, and bowel changes. These carbs, called FODMAPs, are found in some fruits, vegetables, dairy, and grains. In contrast, a gluten-free diet removes all gluten found in wheat, barley, and rye—mainly for those with celiac disease or gluten sensitivity.

While there is overlap (since wheat contains both gluten and the FODMAP fructans), not all gluten-free foods are low in FODMAPs, and vice versa. For example, gluten-free products may use high-FODMAP sweeteners like honey. Always check ingredients and know the unique restrictions of each diet if you combine or follow either.

Can exercise influence IBS symptoms during the diet?

Yes. Regular, moderate exercise helps regulate bowel function, reduces stress, and can ease IBS symptoms such as bloating or constipation. Gentle activities like walking, cycling, yoga, or stretching are often well-tolerated. However, intense workouts or exercising soon after eating can sometimes worsen symptoms for some people. Tracking your exercise, meals, and symptoms can help you learn what works best for you.

How do I handle eating out on a low-FODMAP plan?

Eating out can be challenging but manageable. Start by checking menus online for suitable options, such as plain grilled meats, eggs, vegetables, rice, or potatoes. Avoid dishes described as "creamy," "marinated," or those with onion or garlic. Communicate your dietary needs clearly to staff and request modifications if needed (like sauce on the side). Bringing a small low-FODMAP snack can help if options are limited. Occasional lapses are unlikely to derail your progress and use eating out as a chance to practice flexibility and communication.

What should I do if a food causes delayed symptoms?

IBS symptoms may appear hours or even a day after eating a problematic food. If this happens, review your food and symptom diary for patterns. If a certain food repeatedly coincides with symptoms, try eliminating it for a week and reintroduce it later to confirm if it's a trigger. Avoid making big changes based on a single reaction; a gradual approach helps identify true triggers. If symptoms are severe or confusing, consult a registered dietitian or doctor.

Can low-FODMAP be followed by vegetarians or vegans?

Yes, but it takes careful planning. Many plant proteins like beans and lentils are high in FODMAPs, but small amounts of firm tofu, tempeh, quinoa, and some nuts and seeds are allowed. Ensure adequate nutrition—especially B12, iron, calcium, and omega-3s by using fortified foods or supplements if needed. Cook in batches, plan meals, and consider seeing a dietitian familiar with both plant-based and low-FODMAP diets.

Will gut health suffer long-term on a low-FODMAP diet?

A strict low-FODMAP diet is not meant to be permanent. Some FODMAPs feed healthy gut bacteria, so after 2–4 weeks of elimination, foods are reintroduced to expand your diet while monitoring symptoms. Reintroducing tolerated FODMAPs helps maintain gut health. Eat a variety of allowed fibers and vegetables, and seek professional guidance if you need long-term restrictions.

How do I manage the diet with coexisting food allergies?

Managing both low-FODMAP needs and food allergies is possible with planning. Make a list of all restrictions when shopping and prepping meals. Choose foods that are both low-FODMAP and allergy-safe, read labels carefully, and prepare meals at home when possible. When eating out, clearly explain both needs to staff. If your safe food list becomes very limited, consult a dietitian to ensure you meet your nutritional needs.

References and Helpful Links

Lovell, R., Ford, A.. (2012). Global Prevalence of and Risk Factors for Irritable Bowel Syndrome: A Meta-analysis. Clinical Gastroenterology and Hepatology. https://doi.org/10.1016/j.cgh.2012.02.029

Sperber, A., Bangdiwala, S., Drossman, D. et al.. (2021). Worldwide Prevalence and Burden of Functional Gastrointestinal Disorders, Results of Rome Foundation Global Study. Gastroenterology. https://doi.org/10.1053/j.gastro.2020.04.014

Shepherd, S., Halmos, E., Glance, S.. (2014). The role of FODMAPs in irritable bowel syndrome. Current Opinion in Clinical Nutrition and Metabolic Care. https://doi.org/10.1097/mco.0000000000000116

Drossman, D. (2016). (2016). Schmulson, M. J., & Drossman, D. A. (2017). What is new in Rome IV. Journal of neurogastroenterology and motility, 23(2), 151. https://pmc.ncbi.nlm.nih.gov/articles/PMC5383110/

Halmos, E. (2015). P. et al.. Dietary FODMAP reduction alters the luminal microbiota and reduces colonic fermentation in patients with irritable bowel syndrome. https://gut.bmj.com/content/64/1/93?mod=article_inline

Gibson, P. (2005). R. & Shepherd, S. J.. Personal view: food for thought—western diet and digestive health. https://onlinelibrary.wiley.com/doi/abs/10.1111/j.1365-2036.2005.02506.x

BARRETT, J., GEARRY, R., MUIR, J. et al.. (2010). Dietary poorly absorbed, short‐chain carbohydrates increase delivery of water and fermentable substrates to the proximal colon. Alimentary Pharmacology & Therapeutics. https://doi.org/10.1111/j.1365-2036.2010.04237.x

Staudacher, H. M., Lomer, M. C., Anderson, J. L., Barrett, J. S., Muir, J. G., Irving, P. M., & Whelan, K. (2012). Fermentable carbohydrate restriction reduces luminal bifidobacteria and gastrointestinal symptoms in patients with irritable bowel syndrome. The Journal of nutrition, 142(8), 1510-1518.
https://www.sciencedirect.com/science/article/pii/S0022316622027122

www.ingramcontent.com/pod-product-compliance
Lightning Source LLC
LaVergne TN
LVHW022009200926
848481LV00007B/2300